I0413969

Medicine First Aid Kit:

First Aid Guide How To Use Medicinal Plants and Natural Herbs Remedies

Table of content

Introduction

Wild plants have many medicinal benefits. These plants have been cultivated and harvested from the home gardens for centuries now. Even out in the wild, these plants are present along with their medicinal qualities at your service.

There are certain plants that you must have in your home at your disposal to cure fever and cough at your home without administering any pharmaceutical drugs. You can enjoy certain medicinal benefits of curing cough and fever, and the home remedies recipes that you can make from these plants.

As a matter of fact, small cuts and minor openings on the skin can develop into deep infections when you are out in the wild. These small cuts can cause infections much larger than their size. Abrasions, scrapes, and minor cuts become a matter of course if you are wandering out there in the wild.

Our grandparents always turned to spices and herbs to ward off these common diseases. You can cure dozens of common ailments with medicinal plants. If you are facing any specific health conditions or have an allergy to certain herbs then you must consult your practitioner before starting using these home remedies.

Chapter 01: Life Saver Plants in the Wilderness

Wild plants have many medicinal benefits. These plants have been cultivated and harvested from the home gardens for centuries now. Using the healing powers of these plants represents a healthier way of living in the modern times. However, these plants can never take the place of regular medical care, but they provide you the sense of security in any emergency that you are not alone, and life saver is sitting in your garden bed for you all the time. Even out in the wild, these plants are present along with their medicinal qualities at your service.

Here, in this chapter, we are discussing some of the life saver plants which can provide you great first aid out in the wild;

Birch:

Barks of birch are accessible in any wild area. They have analgesic qualities especially the sweet birch barks are abundant with it if they have enough salicylates. You can also make a delicious tea by scrapping 1 to 2 grams of bark from the sweet birch twigs and boiling it with about 7 ounces of water. But it is important to consume as per the recommended doses only otherwise you can suffer tinnitus, nausea, or upset stomach. You must stop drinking it as soon as any of these reactions start developing in your body. However, a higher intake of 240 mg per day of salicin has been proven to be more useful for treating pain through scientific research.

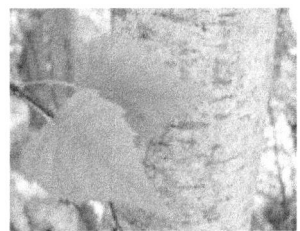

Jewelweed:

It is common for you to come into contact with sumac, oak, or poison ivy out in the wild. In such a scenario, you must locate and make a paste by crushing its purplish, juicy stalk. Apply this paste all over the affected area of your body. Let it dry for two minutes. Afterward, rinse it off with clean water. You will have little to no reaction if you can get this treatment within thirty to forty-five minutes of your body's contact with the poison ivy. You can still have its relieving benefits by using it as a wash if you don't find it within the time. If you are experiencing itch and blisters on your skin, then it shows that the contact with poison ivy was made yesterday, in such a case, jewelweed will help you relief the pain.

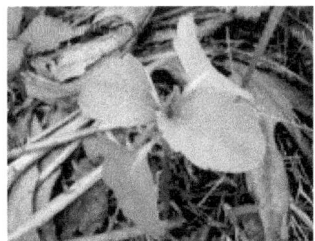

Black Walnut:

These walnuts have green husks. These husks are of a significant medicinal value in the folk medicine. If you want to have a sip of a parasite expelling tea out in the wild, then boil one tablespoon of dried green husks of black walnuts with one cup of hot water. The taste is going to be horrible! But you don't need to take the full cup at one time, sip it during the whole of the day, and repeat this process for seven days consecutively. You can also use the fresh green husks of the black walnuts. They have great antiseptic properties and replace the regular tincture iodine in the wild for you.

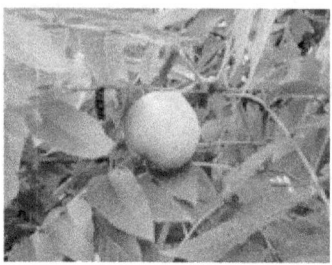

Elderberry:

You can treat wounds with it. You can also take it orally to treat cold, flu, and other respiratory illnesses. The chemical in it can also relief the swelling of the mucous membranes. It also relieves nasal congestion. It contains anticancer, antiviral, and anti-inflammatory properties. You can consume it in the form of wine or jam in your house. Remember that raw elderberries can have a little toxic effect on your body. Also, they can have drug interactions with immune system-suppressing drugs, theophylline, laxatives, chemotherapy, diabetes medications, and diuretics.

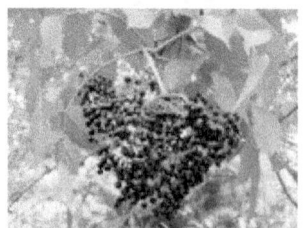

Echinacea:

Consuming Echinacea products on the appearance of the initial symptoms of a cold can reduce its duration and effect in adults. The products also significantly impact the vaginal yeast infections. Applying medicated cream to the affected body part is pertinent. Its plant compounds attack the yeast and other fungi. It drops the reoccurring chance of the infection by 16%.

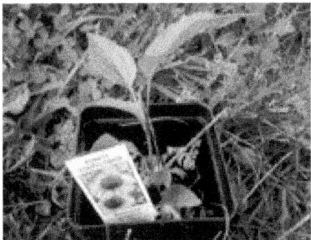

Willow:

You can make an effective astringent by boiling ten to twelve leaves of weeping willow with one cup of water. Dip a cloth in it and apply directly on the ulcers, carbuncles, and abscesses in the absence of any other medical treatment. If you want an anti-diarrhea drink out in the wild, soak fresh bark (without twigs) in a cup of warm water, and sip it.

One of its prominent family members is black willow. It has anti-inflammatory and pain-relieving effects due to the presence of salicin in it. It relieves fever as well.

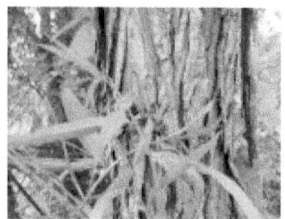

Dandelion:

It is a general gall bladder/liver tonic. Mix one tablespoon of the dried root with one cup water to make a tea for stimulating digestion. You can use it three times a day. You can make its solution with alcohol as well.

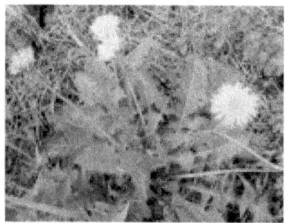

Plantain:

You can locate in any garden beds, fields, and lawns. It is a humble weed with many medicinal benefits. Although it is not strong enough to fight a snake's venom, applying its paste on venomous bites and stings of scorpions, wasps, bees, and some other pain inducing creatures has a great effect. You need to keep on replacing the paste as it dries out on the bite.

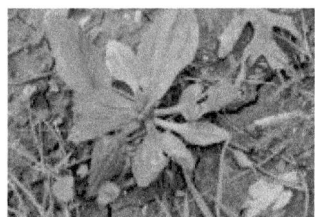

Burdock:

It is an excellent liver tonic. It is also helpful in purifying the body and blood. You can use both of its leaves and roots. You can also get rid of the acne with it. It has significant on other skin conditions like eczema, etc. as well if you consume ten to twenty drops of its tincture by mixing its dried leaves with alcohol.

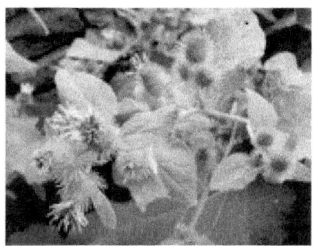

Chapter 02: Medicinal Plants for Cough and Fever

There are certain plants that you must have in your home at your disposal to cure fever and cough at your home without administering any pharmaceutical drugs. These plants include oregano, lemon, barley, mint, eucalyptus, etc. Having knowledge about these plants will help you to have first aid treatment out in the wild as well.

In this chapter, we will discuss some of the plants with medicinal benefits of a curing cough and fever, and the home remedies recipes that you can make from these plants. Let's read together!

Oregano:

It is good for cold and cough relief. Make a solution by boiling one cup of fresh leaves with three cups of water. Keep this solution in a bottle or jug, and drink half a cup three times a day. Keep this routine for one week.

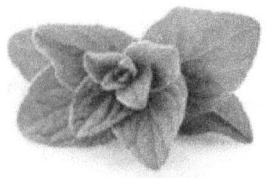

Barley:

It is helpful in reducing fever and hydrating the body. Make a solution of two tablespoons of barley water with two liters of water and boil it until half of the solution is vaporized. Add one tablespoon of lemon juice. Sip two glasses of this solution per day.

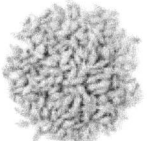

Mint:

It has a significant medicinal value as it reduces the fever by increasing the sweating in a human body. You can take it through infusing a tablespoon of dried mint. Take two to three cups for a couple of days.

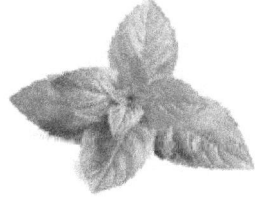

Hibiscus:

It is great to relief fever and cough. Infuse one teaspoon of dried hibiscus leaves in one cup of water. Consume this solution for a couple of days.

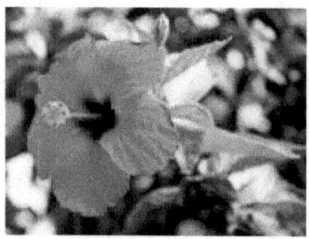

Eucalyptus:

Eucalyptus essential oil has anti-fever properties. You do not need to drink but to add a few drops of its oil on a wet cloth and apply on the skin to reduce the fever.

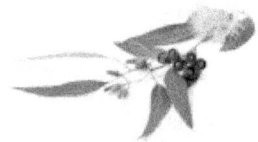

Violet:

This plant produces the violet color of flowers. These flowers have high anti-fever properties. Infuse a tablespoon of the dried flowers in a liter of water. Consume two to three cups of this solution every day to reduce the body temperature.

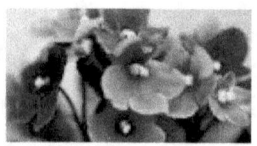

Thyme:

It reduces the effects of an infection by reducing the fever as it contains high antiseptic properties. You can also use it to relief your sore throat especially if it is a case of angina. Infuse a tablespoon of the dried flowers of thyme in a cup of water. Take three to four cups a day to relief the pain.

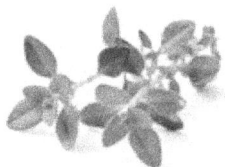

Elderberry:

You can take it orally to treat cold, flu, and other respiratory illnesses. It also relieves nasal congestion. It contains anticancer, antiviral, and anti-inflammatory properties. You can consume it in the form of wine or jam in your house.

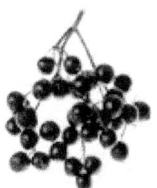

Ginger:

This plant is gorgeous with antibacterial and antiviral properties. It eliminates the effects of infections such as fever, cold, and influenza. Infuse a teaspoon of its dried root in a cup of water. Consume two to three cups per day for a week. You can also add a teaspoon of lemon juice per cup to enhance its medicinal value.

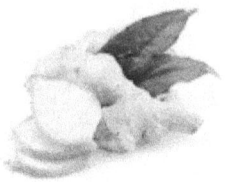

Coffee:

Coffee leaves have anti-fever properties. You can consume them by making water or milk solution.

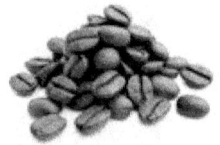

Pumpkin:

Everyone loves pumpkins. Their leaves are rich in anti-fever properties. You can make pumpkin leaves tea by boiling one and a half cup of the leaves in one liter of water. Let the solution stand for one hour. Consume three to four cups a day.

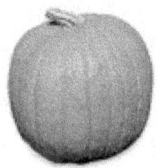

Willow:

All members of willow family contain anti-fever properties. You can consume it in the form of tea.

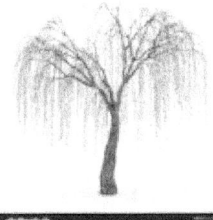

Meadowsweet:

This plant has high anti-fever properties. Infuse one teaspoon of its flowers in a couple of cups of water. Consume two to three cups a day.

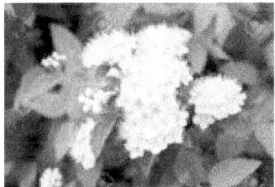

Vervain:

Reducing fever in a human body is good. Infuse a teaspoon of the dried plant in a cup of water. Consume two to three cups of this infusion in a day.

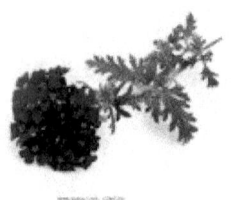

Soursop or Guanabana:

The leaves of this plant have antipyretic, sleep-inducing, and tranquilizing properties. You can consume it in the fever to relax your body and get a good sleep.

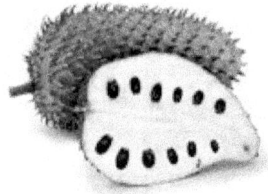

Panikoorka:

It is an ayurvedic herb. Its leaves have significant anti-fever, anti-cold, and cough-reducing properties. It is also perfect for children. It relieves chest congestion, nasal congestion, sore throat, fever, cold, and cough. Make a solution of two to three drops of the juice of its leaves in a cup of water and consume one cup per day for a week.

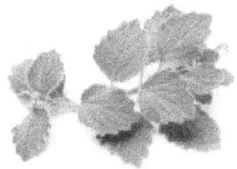

Tulsi:

You can chew its leaves to relief a sore throat, flu, and cough. Make its tea by boiling five to six fresh basil leaves in a cup of water. Consume this tea two to three times a day.

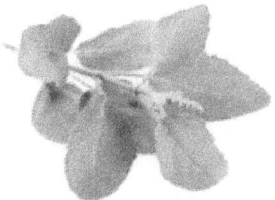

Henna:

Leaves of this plant have great medicinal values. However, its seeds have significant anti-fever properties. You can consume it as a tea.

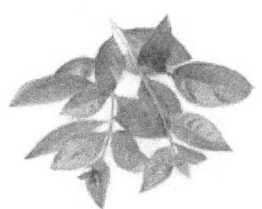

Neem:

It is a great plant. You can use every part of this plant for their great medicinal benefits. Its bark has analgesic properties. It reduces fever in a human body.

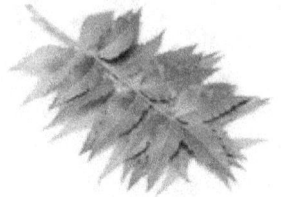

Bidens Pilosa:

This plant has high anti-fever properties. Consume its tea to minimize the temperature of a human body.

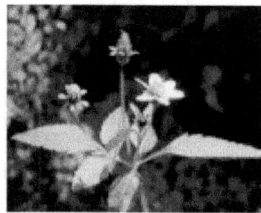

Sunflower:

In addition to adding beauty to the landscape of your garden by its beautiful yellow flowers, this plant has anti-fever properties. You can consume it in the form of tea.

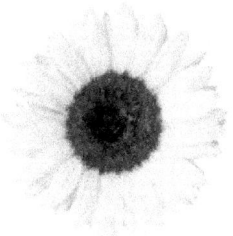

Catnip:

It's effective to reduce fever because it increases the rate of sweating in a human body. Consume its tea two to three times a day.

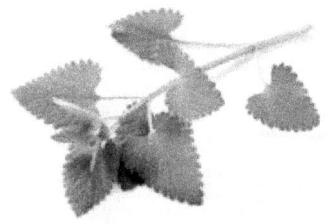

Chapter 03: Natural Antiseptics in the Wilderness

Abrasions, scrapes, and minor cuts become a matter of course if you are wandering out there in the wild. These small cuts can cause infections much larger than their size. As a matter of fact, small cuts and minor openings on the skin can develop into deep infections when you are out in the wild. Nature has a habit of balancing out every action. Therefore, many great plants with enormous medicinal values are found everywhere on this beautiful planet. All you need is the knowledge so that you can use them as a first aid in the absence of any other medical treatment.

In this chapter, we will discuss some of the wild plants and herbs with great antiseptic values. Let's read together!

Garlic:

If you get a cut or wound, the first step you should take is to stop the bleeding. You must put pressure on the injury to stop it either by your hand or more preferably with a clean cloth. After you have succeeded in stopping the bleeding, you must clean and disinfect the body area. One of the great antiseptics that you found in the wild is garlic. Fresh garlic has both antiviral and antibacterial properties. It is pertinent to use fresh garlic as older bulbs lose their medicinal values over time. Cut a new piece of garlic, chop or crush it, and rub on the wound.

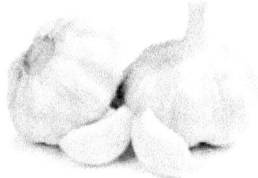

Tea Tree Oil:

This essential oil is extracted from the leaves of a plant of tea tree. It has excellent antiseptic properties. You can apply it topically on the wound to disinfect the skin patch. It kills microbial infections in seconds. Use this oil to the injured skin before dressing it to avoid the harmful diseases. Don't take it orally. It is toxic for human this way.

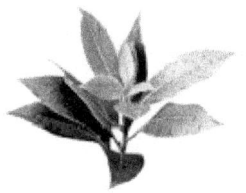

Honey:

Honey is the most proven and tested antiseptic available out there in the wild. It exhibits antiseptic properties against a broad spectrum of bacteria. It also helps the wounds and cuts on skin to heal faster. It maintains a moist environment around the injured patch of the skin as well. You must always wrap the skin area with a clean cloth after applying honey so that dirt and debris do not get stuck in it. Honey contains high sugar content. Therefore, you must expect bears, dogs, and ants getting attracted to you out in the wild!

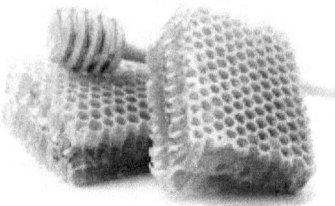

Aloe Vera Juice:

Aloe Vera has excellent dermatological properties. It also increases the rate of healing of the human skin. It has significant antibacterial properties. Therefore, you can use it on your wound to kill the bacteria and reducing the healing time.

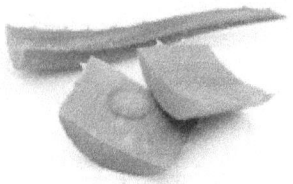

Burdock:

Every part of this plant contains high values of antiseptic properties. It has antibacterial compounds that fight the microbial on the infected part of the skin and disinfect it to prevent any future harmful infection. It is an excellent liver tonic. It is also helpful in purifying the body and blood. You can use both of its leaves and roots. You can also get rid of the acne with it.

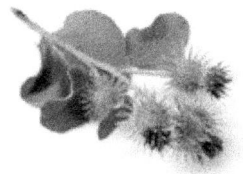

Peppermint:

It is a plant with a high level of antibacterial components. It fights infections. You can apply its essential oil on the wound. Menthol is a germ killer. You can also add a few drops of peppermint essential oil in boiling water to give yourself a soothing steam. It is an existing plant, so you don't even need to take a towel to your head to take the steam. But be careful and do not take your eyes or nose too close to the oil since you can only apply it externally.

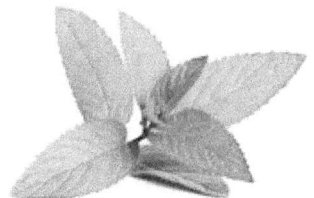

Thyme:

It is another great disinfectant. It has high antibacterial components. It reduces the effects of an infection by reducing the fever as it contains high antiseptic properties. It is antiparasitic, antispasmodic, antiseptic, antibacterial, and an excellent tonic as well.

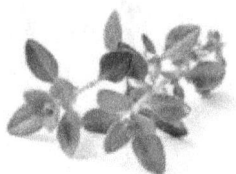

Calendula:

It is a vulnerary agent. It has healing powers. It is slightly antimicrobial and anti-inflammatory. You can use it topically to heal internally infected mucous membranes, skin infections, and abrasions.

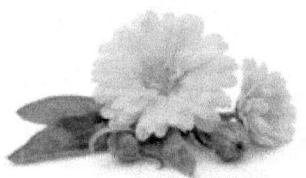

Chamomile:

It contains awesome relaxation properties. Its dried flowers contain flavonoids and terpenoids. You can make a chamomile flower press for your wound. It reduces the healing time.

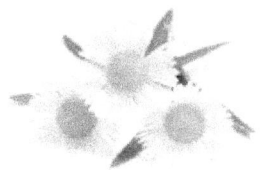

Potato:

These roots have a gravitational pull which enhances their medicinal value. They can draw out infection from any cut, abscess, or wound on your skin. Take a potato and shred it. Place it on the wound. Keep on replacing it every three to four hours. It reduces inflammation as well. Thus, there remains no chance of infection in the skin.

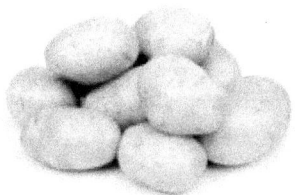

Lavender:

Lavender is known for producing hasty tissue regeneration. It does this miracle without any scarring on your skin. You can use to reduce the healing time of your wound as well. You can use it topically by applying two to four drops of its essential oil on the wound for two to three times a day.

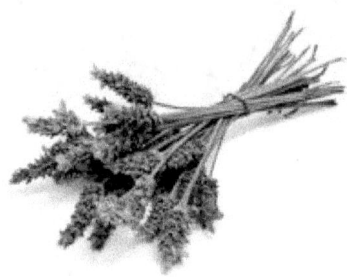

Goldenseal:

This plant has excellent astringent and antiseptic properties. You can use it to heal stings, bites, infections, wounds, and cuts. You can also consume it to treat inflammation of the intestinal tract and stomach, and sinus infections. It contains hydrastine and berberine which help it fight and destroy many kinds of viral and bacterial infections. You can use its ointment on your skin as well.

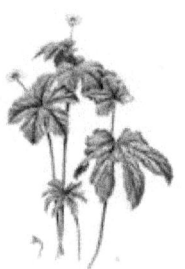

Chapter 04: Natural Remedies for Common Ailments

You can cure dozens of common ailments with medicinal plants. Our grandparents always turned to spices and herbs to ward off these common diseases. So, you can skip the trip to the drugstore. The help is sitting right in front of you, in your kitchen cabinet. These time-tested remedies are proven effective and safe.

Note: if you are facing any specific health conditions or have an allergy to certain herbs then you must consult your practitioner before starting using these home remedies.

In this chapter, we are going to discuss some of the miraculous home remedies to cure the common, regular ailments. Let's read together!

Urinary Tract Infection:

It is a common infection. Overall, women get infected with it more than the men. The best home remedy to cure a UTI is to use cranberry juice. You can also use dried berries and their extract. They have the same impact of preventing the bacteria from sticking to and spreading in the gall bladder. You must, at least, consume three cups of the juice (mixed with apple juice) in a day. But it is pertinent to keep it unsweetened. You can also eat a cup of dried berries a day alternatively.

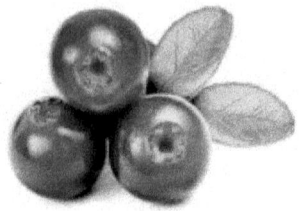

Bruises:

If you are a person who is prone to bumping into doors and side-tables then this fork remedy is soon becoming your new best friend. Cut a lemon in half and rub it directly on the bruise. It will speed up the healing process. Don't apply on broken skin or cuts.

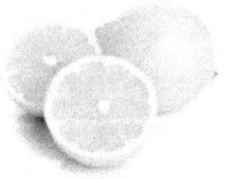

Joint Pain and Arthritis:

If you suffer from joint pain or arthritis then you must give a try to turmeric. It has an active ingredient curcumin which is proven to be reducing joint pains in the human body. It also contains anti-inflammatory properties. You can use it as a part of your daily food such as vegetables, stir-fries, sauces, and soups.

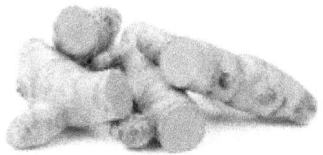

Cancer Prevention:

According to the U.S Department of Agriculture, many herbs are a great source of providing cancer-preventive antioxidants to our bodies. Oregano, cloves, and cinnamon have high antioxidant capacities. Green tea is helpful in reducing the chances of cancer in skin, stomach, breast, and lungs.

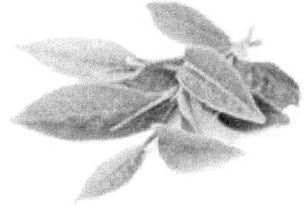

Nausea:

You can effectively and safely relief nausea with ginger. It is also helpful in preventing motion sickness. You can consume it in the form of a tea by boiling two teaspoons of freshly grated ginger in water for ten minutes.

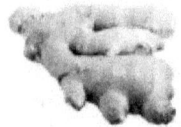

Digestion:

Many people suffer from digestion issues. It is a common thing. Many culinary herbs are helpful in relieving gas and bloating. You must consume one to two cups of peppermint tea for general upset stomach or indigestion. The chewing half teaspoon of dill seeds, caraway, or fennel relieves the gas.

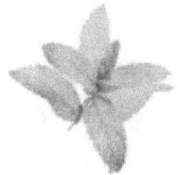

Sinus Problems:

If you are suffering from painful and clogged sinuses then you must give a try to this spicy mixture. Combine one teaspoon of lemon juice, a one-fourth teaspoon of cayenne powder, one teaspoon of freshly chopped garlic, and one cup tomato juice. Consume it in several hours. Warm up every time.

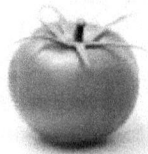

Coughs:

Thyme contains great expectorant properties. If you are facing bronchitis, sore throat, congestion, or a cough then using thyme is a great choice for you. It also contains strong antimicrobial properties. Boil one teaspoon of dried leaves of thyme in one cup of water for ten to twelve minutes and sip the tea. You can drink up to three cups of this tea in a day.

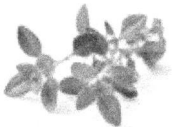

Boost Your Immunity:

Several medicinal plants are great in boosting the immunity system of a human body. Garlic is a potent antioxidant. It fights cancer and enhances the capacity of the immunity system. Green tea is also rich in antioxidant components. You can drink several cups of its tea daily. Echinacea contains immune-stimulating constituents as well.

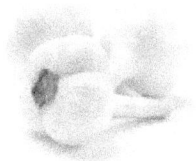

High Blood Sugar:

Cinnamon can help reduce the level of sugar in the human blood. You can use it in regular cooking or consume it in the form of tea. Boil half teaspoon of cinnamon powder in one cup of water to make the tea. Cover the drink for ten minutes. You can consume up to three cups of this per day.

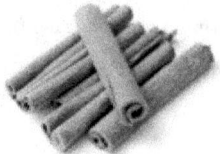

High Cholesterol and Heart Health:

Garlic contains miraculous cholesterol controlling capacities. It also reduces the risks of heart attack and heart diseases. You can consume in raw form up to one clove per day. It also reduces the LDL cholesterol levels in a human body.

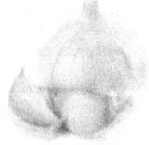

Common Cold:

You can reduce the harshness of common cold with garlic soup. Consuming one glass of lemon juice per day will increase the level of your body resistance against the cold as well. Onion juice is also helpful in preventing the cold. Don't forget to drink plenty of water, around six to eight glasses per day.

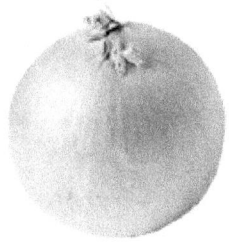

Fever Blisters:

If you are experiencing blisters on your skin due to any reason, apply petroleum jelly on them. Apply cold compress on the affected patch of the skin after applying this jelly. Avoid consuming chocolate and nuts as well.

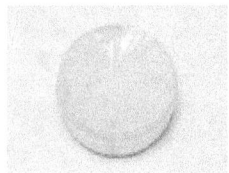

Sore Throat:

Mix honey, lemon juice, and hot water and consume this tea to relief your sore throat. Avoid eating chilies and other hot spices. You can also consume marshmallows.

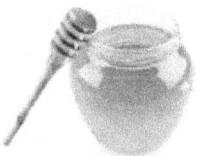

Heartburn:

If you are suffering from heartburn, eat bananas. They are antacid. Fresh ginger is also helpful in reducing heartburn. You can add it in your food, or eat it raw. Another option is to make its tea. You can take up to three cups of this tea in a day.

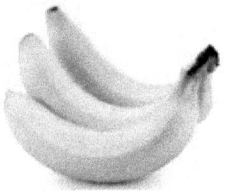

Chapter 05: Precautions to Use Medicinal Plants and Natural Herbs

Herbal plants contain great healing powers. They are known to do the miracles without any side effects. These medicinal plants do not contain any chemical, therefore, they do not harm human body the other commercial products would. It is the main difference between the market products and the herbal remedies. These herbal treatments even come with a lot of minerals and vitamins. These goodies add energy in our bodies and protect us from different kinds of ailments. They are also more affordable in comparison to other products.

Even with all these miraculous properties and abilities, you must observe some cautions and safety methods while using these little bundles of great health values. Remember that things lose their good values if you use them in an excess amount. Similarly, an overdose of a natural remedy will worsen the health scenario for you.

In this chapter, we are discussing some precautions and safety measures that you must adopt while enjoying the health benefits of the natural herbs and medicinal plants. Let's read together!

General Considerations:

These herbal products are commonly safe to use but using them without proper guidance can be fatal or dangerous for you. Most of these herbal formulae consist of essential oils and using them in raw form and excess amounts can result in certain side effects.

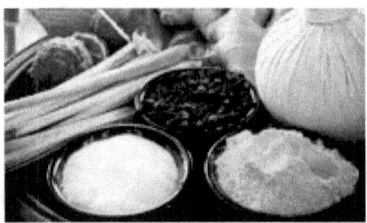

Most of the people use natural products as much as they can because these are natural, right?! So, you can use it freely. But this is not the right scenario. You must never use anything in excess of the prescribed amount.

Sometimes the natural herbs are grown using heavy doses of chemicals in the field. These chemicals have their impact on the constituency of the herbs and plants, therefore, natural products along with their handful of effective results have some little side effects too. Certain other precaution must also be kept in mind when using medicinal plants and natural herbs.

Precautions when Using Chamomile:

Most the people in this world have a fairly high tolerance for chamomile herb and they can enjoy two to three cups of its tea on any particular day. However, many people are allergic to it. Therefore, they cannot consume this tea over an extended period. It is pertinent to use this herb well within the recommended dose.

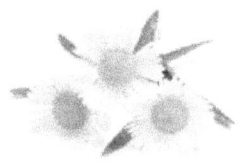

Precautions with Therapeutic Herbal Combinations:

As a general piece of advice, any herbal combination in therapeutic doses must not be taken consecutively for more than twelve weeks unless you are professionally advised after complete check to continue the process. This safety measure is adopted because a human body becomes addicted and habitual to these natural scents within days. Also, certain systems in a human body can suffer an irritant effect due to the chemicals of certain plants under the cumulative exposure. You must also consult a health adviser if the accepted results are not shown within twelve weeks of the therapy.

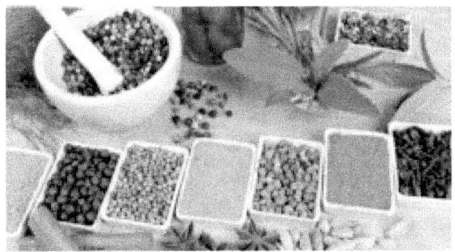

Precautions in Consuming Stimulant Herbs:

You must consume all kinds of stimulant herbs early in the morning. It is not ideal to such a herb before going to bed. Uterus stimulating herbs are good for delaying menstruation cycle but you must avoid taking it during the pregnancy.

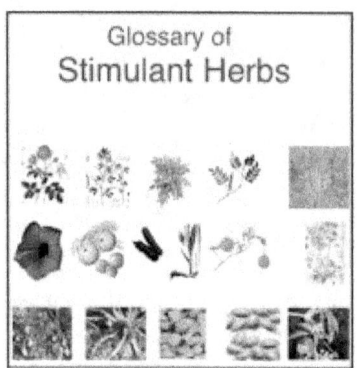

Precautions with Black Cohosh:

Although, it happens in rare cases but black cohosh can disturb the regular liver activities in your stomach. If you are already experiencing any kind of liver issues and problems then it is recommendable to consult your doctor before starting to use this herb. Also, go to your health advisory if you start to experiencing some sort of problems in your body whilst the use.

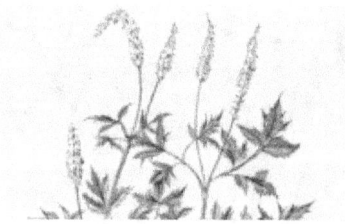

Precautions in Taking Herbs During Pregnancy:

You must avoid taking uterus stimulating herbs such as strong laxatives, emmenagogues, and abortifacients during all stages of pregnancy. You must also not consume ground ivy, gravel root, borage, aloe vera, angelica root, avens, and beth root when pregnant. You can consume basil, aniseed, cinnamon, and fenugreek but only in smart doses.

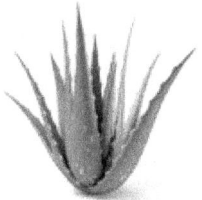

Contraindications During Lactation:

If you are a mother and breastfeeding your children then you must avoid consuming basil, bayberry, blue cohosh, calamus root, and comfrey. However, you can consume garlic in small doses only.

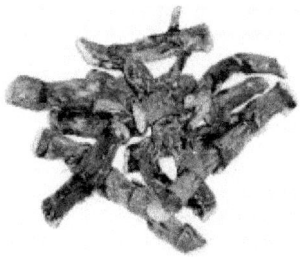

These medicinal plants and natural herbs can never take the place of regular medical care, but they provide you the sense of security in any emergency that you are not alone, and life saver is sitting in your garden bed for you all the time. Nature has a habit of balancing out every action. Therefore, many great plants with enormous medicinal values are found everywhere on this beautiful planet.

All you need is the knowledge so that you can use them as a first aid in the absence of any other medical treatment. Remember that things lose their good values if you use them in an excess amount. Similarly, an overdose of a natural remedy will worsen the health scenario for you. If you are facing any specific health conditions or have an allergy to certain herbs then you must consult your practitioner before starting using these home remedies.

Conclusion

Using the healing powers of these plants represents a healthier way of living in the modern times. Even out in the wild, these plants are present along with their medicinal qualities at your service.

There are certain plants that you must have in your home at your disposal such as oregano, lemon, barley, mint, eucalyptus, etc. Nature has a habit of balancing out every action. Therefore, many great plants with enormous medicinal values are found everywhere on this beautiful planet.

These medicinal plants help the wounds and cuts on skin to heal faster. They contain excellent dermatological properties. They have antibacterial compounds that fight the microbial on the infected part of the skin and disinfect it to prevent any future harmful infection.

These natural herbs also have high level of antibacterial components as well as awesome relaxation properties. They reduce the healing time.

FREE Bonus Reminder

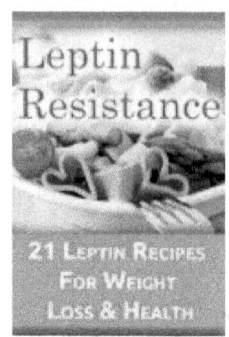

If you have not grabbed it yet, please go ahead and download your special bonus report *"Leptin Resistance. 21 Leptin Recipes For Weight Loss & Healthy Living"*.

Simply Click the Button Below

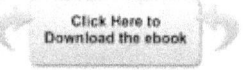

OR **Go to This Page**

http://easyweightlossway.com/free/

BONUS #2: More Free & Discounted Books

Do you want to receive more Free & Discounted Books?

We have a mailing list where we send out our new Books when they go free or with a discount on Kindle. Click on the link below to sign up for Free & Discount Book Promotions.

=> Sign Up for Free & Discount Book Promotions <=

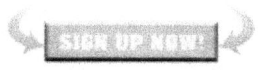

OR Go to this URL

http://zbit.ly/1WBb1Ek

www.ingramcontent.com/pod-product-compliance
Lightning Source LLC
Chambersburg PA
CBHW071145280526
45787CB00003B/1418